PARENTING TEENAGERS WITH ADHD

NURTURING ADOLESCENCE: EMPOWERING TEENS WITH ADHD FOR SUCCESS

MICHAEL E. HOWELL

Preface:

Raising an adolescent can be both an amazing and challenging experience in a world that sometimes appears to advance at an alarming rate. Imagine having ADHD and navigating the choppy seas of puberty at the same time. Even when confronted with particular challenges, it is our deep obligation as parents to nurture, mentor, and empower our kids. "Parenting Teenagers with ADHD: Nurturing Adolescence" takes shape in this environment.

This book was inspired by the conviction that, despite the difficulties they may encounter, every adolescent deserves the chance to develop.

We are aware of the everyday struggles, irritations, and periods of extreme tiredness associated with raising an ADHD-affected adolescent. In addition to the mayhem, there is a wealth of love, resiliency, and unrealized potential that is just waiting to be found.

We welcome you to investigate the complex nature of ADHD and its effects on youth as we begin this adventure together. Through these pages, we will go into the depths of comprehension, empathy, and practical techniques to support our kids as they not only cope but also develop into self-assured, prosperous adults.

We strive to provide you with a thorough manual that addresses the particular requirements of kids with ADHD by drawing on a variety of research, expert insights, and personal experiences. We will examine useful strategies and sympathetic methods that may change adolescence from a turbulent time to one of development and self-discovery, from encouraging open communication and creating healthy relationships to overcoming scholastic hurdles and growing self-esteem.

We also understand that each adolescent is a unique person and that what works for one may not necessarily work for another. Therefore, we urge you to modify and customize the advice provided on these pages to fit the particular requirements, aptitudes, and interests of your adolescent. Never forget that there is a community of parents, educators, and professionals willing to assist you and provide their knowledge. You are not alone in this path. Our common objective is to give our ADHD-affected kids the confidence, resiliency, and bravery to embrace their talents. Let's rewrite the history of ADHD together, replacing stigmas with understanding, restrictions with limitless opportunities, and struggles with victories.

May this book be a beacon of hope, showing the way to fostering adolescence and equipping our extraordinary teens with ADHD for success throughout their lives?

With love and steadfast commitment.

CONTENTS

PART I: UNDERSTANDING ADHD AND ADOLESCENCE

CHAPTER 1: UNRAVELING ADHD IN ADOLESCENCE

Neurodevelopmental problem Attention Deficit Hyperactivity disorder (ADHD) affects people of all ages, although adolescence is when it often manifests and poses special difficulties. Understanding and treating ADHD becomes essential for teens' general well-being and achievement as they go through considerable physical, cognitive, and emotional changes. This article seeks to clarify the difficulties of ADHD in adolescence and investigate methods for determining its effects.

Chronic patterns of impulsivity, hyperactivity, and inattention that affect everyday functioning and academic achievement are hallmarks of ADHD. Teenagers may have extra challenges as a result of the symptoms of ADHD developing or becoming more noticeable throughout puberty. Teenagers with ADHD often struggle with developing organizational skills, managing their time, paying attention in class, and reining in impulsive behaviors. These difficulties may cause poor self-esteem, strained relationships with family and friends, academic underachievement, and a higher chance of participating in hazardous activities.

The increasing pressures and expectations put on teens throughout adolescence may contribute to ADHD symptoms being more pronounced during this period.

A more demanding academic burden, more courses, extracurricular activities, and increased social demands come with the move to high school. These elements may overwhelm those who have ADHD, making it harder for them to concentrate, prioritize work, and keep to their schedules. ADHD symptoms may also be complicated by hormonal changes that occur throughout puberty, which can have an impact on mood and emotional control.

Effective intervention requires early detection and diagnosis of ADHD in adolescents. Teenagers with ADHD might be difficult to diagnose since their symptoms can resemble normal adolescent behavior or mood problems like despair or anxiety. In particular, if the adolescent makes up for their inattentiveness by exerting more effort or depending on outside assistance, the symptoms of inattentiveness may go unnoticed.

The signs and symptoms of ADHD, such as forgetfulness, trouble organizing activities, an inability to maintain attention, excessive fidgeting, impulsivity, and poor time management, must be recognized by parents, teachers, and healthcare professionals..When ADHD is discovered in adolescence, a thorough approach to care and support is crucial. Teenagers may manage their ADHD symptoms to a great extent by using a variety of methods that include medication, psychoeducation, behavioral interventions, and support from parents, teachers, and mental health specialists.

A medical expert may recommend medication, such as stimulant or non-stimulant drugs, to assist manage attention and impulsive control. These drugs balance neurotransmitters in the brain, but their usage should always be closely watched and altered while being overseen by a medical practitioner.

Teenagers with ADHD need psychoeducation to help them understand their illness and create coping mechanisms for its difficulties. Adolescents' feelings of control and self-assurance may be improved by educating them about ADHD, how it affects their everyday life, and how to advocate for themselves. Psychoeducation may also entail cultivating empathy and establishing a supportive atmosphere while teaching parents, teachers, and peers about ADHD.

Adolescents with ADHD are taught practical strategies to help with organization, time management, and study habits as part of behavioral therapies. These therapies often entail establishing precise objectives, establishing organized routines, using visual aids, and using tools for organizing like planners or digital applications.

In addition to treating ADHD, cognitive-behavioral therapy (CBT) may help with comorbid illnesses including depression or anxiety. In addition to receiving expert assistance, parents and instructors are crucial in assisting teenagers with ADHD in overcoming their difficulties. For the adolescent to feel more confident and motivated, open communication, structure, consistency, realistic expectations, and tiny victories may all be very helpful. For kids with ADHD, the playing field may be leveled by working with teachers to offer accommodations like extra time for tasks or preferred seating in the classroom.

Creating a welcoming and inclusive social climate is also important. It is essential for young people with ADHD. Peers who tolerate and comprehend people with ADHD may be a beneficial support system and enhance a teen's general well-being.

Reducing stigma and fostering acceptance among peers may help create a more welcoming learning environment in schools.

A multifaceted strategy that takes into account the particular difficulties and developmental transitions that teens experience is necessary to unravel ADHD in adolescence. Adolescents with ADHD may learn techniques to control their symptoms, gain resilience, and succeed academically, socially, and emotionally by combining medication, psychoeducation, behavioral interventions, and support from parents, teachers, and mental health experts. As they enter adulthood, people with ADHD may have productive lives and realize their full potential with the correct support and understanding.

The Impact of ADHD on Teenagers

Millions of people worldwide, including a sizable proportion of teens, are affected by Attention Deficit Hyperactivity disorder (ADHD), a neurodevelopmental illness. Academic performance, social connections, emotional health, and general development may all be significantly impacted by ADHD in adolescence. To provide the right assistance and therapies to help teens with ADHD successfully navigate these issues, it is essential to understand the unique challenges they confront.

One area where the effects of ADHD on teens are most noticeable is academic performance. Teenagers with ADHD often struggle to stay focused, organize their chores, manage their time, and finish their projects. Lower grades, incomplete or missing assignments, and difficulty keeping up with the academic requirements of school may all be consequences of these issues. Teenagers with ADHD may therefore feel frustrated, like they are failing in school, and have lower self-esteem. The long-term effects of the academic challenges may have an impact on the students' opportunities for further education and employment.

ADHD in adolescents may also have an impact on social relationships. Peer connections and social approval take on more significance throughout adolescence. Teenagers with ADHD, however, may display impulsive conduct, have trouble reading social signs, and have trouble controlling their impulses, which may cause social challenges. They could struggle to manage their emotions, take turns in talks, and follow social standards, which can cause strained friendships and social isolation. Their general well-being and sense of self-worth may be further impacted by their lack of social relationships and rejection.

Adolescents with ADHD may also struggle emotionally and psychologically. Anxiety and sadness are two more mental health problems that often co-occur with ADHD. Stress levels might rise and emotional dysregulation can occur as a result of ADHD sufferers' ongoing battles to live up to expectations, control symptoms, and deal with everyday difficulties. The emotional and psychological effects on teens are further exacerbated by the impulsivity and inattention that are symptoms of ADHD, which may also result in impulsive decision-making and risk-taking behaviors.

The difficulties associated with ADHD may have a substantial impact on self-esteem and confidence. Teenagers with ADHD can contrast themselves with their friends, seeing how they struggle to keep up, remain organized, or finish chores. Feelings of inadequacy, annoyance, and self-doubt may result from this.

Furthermore, criticism of their conduct or academic performance from classmates, parents, or instructors may further erode their self-esteem. For teens with ADHD to build resilience and a good self-image, support and encouragement are essential.

Teenagers with ADHD have effects that go beyond their own lives and affect their family relationships as well. To support their child's academic development, manage their conduct, and attend to their emotional needs, parents of teens with ADHD often encounter special problems. Conflict, guilt, and irritation may sometimes result from familial pressure and stress. To successfully help their adolescent and preserve a harmonious home life, parents must seek out assistance and information regarding ADHD.

Despite the difficulties, it's important to keep in mind that ADHD does not entirely determine a teen's personality or potential.

Teenagers with ADHD are capable of flourishing and reaching their full potential with the right therapies, support, and understanding. Teenagers may manage their symptoms and overcome the difficulties linked to ADHD with significant help from early detection, diagnosis, and a thorough treatment plan that may include medication, counseling, educational accommodations, and behavioral interventions.

Additionally, fostering a welcoming and encouraging atmosphere in communities and schools may significantly lessen the effects of ADHD on youth. Teaching others about ADHD may increase empathy, lessen stigma, and create a supportive network for youth with the condition. Teens with ADHD may have severe effects in a variety of facets of their life. ADHD may have an impact on a variety of areas, including social interaction, mental health, and family relationships. Recognizing and comprehending the difficulties that come with Providing the right support and therapies for teens with ADHD is essential for their success. Teenagers with ADHD may overcome challenges, develop coping skills, and lead happy, fulfilled lives with the correct support structure and therapies in place.

Embracing their Potential and Strengths

Attention deficit hyperactivity disorder (ADHD) is often accompanied by obstacles and problems. However, it's equally crucial to acknowledge and capitalize on the abilities and assets that adolescents with ADHD have. We can provide kids with the tools they need to overcome challenges, develop resilience, and make great contributions to society by concentrating on their strengths.

The following are some important areas where adolescents with ADHD often exhibit extraordinary potential and strengths:

1. _inventiveness_: Many adolescents with ADHD exhibit extraordinary inventiveness. Their capacity to think creatively, integrate seemingly unrelated ideas, and approach issues from several perspectives may result in original and inventive solutions. Their creative thinking may be a useful tool in a variety of fields, including the arts, literature, and problem-solving.

2. _Hyperfocus_: People with ADHD may also experience hyperfocus, which is an intense concentration on things that pique their interest, even while they have trouble maintaining attention. Teenagers with ADHD may display amazing attention and productivity when they discover a topic or activity they are enthusiastic about.
Utilizing this hyperfocus may result in remarkable accomplishments in fields of personal interest.

3. _Energy and excitement_: Adhd teens often have a lot of energy and excitement. While it

could be difficult for them to direct this energy effectively, when it is, it can produce extraordinary determination, tenacity, and enthusiasm for life. Their energy may spread and motivate others around them.

4. <u>*Unconventional Thinking*</u>: People with ADHD often have unorthodox thought processes and original viewpoints. Teenagers with ADHD may provide unique perspectives, see connections that others might miss, and generate original thoughts. Their capacity to address issues outside of the box may result in innovations and breakthroughs.

5. *Resilience and Adaptability*: To manage ADHD, one must constantly adjust and be resilient in the face of difficulties. Teenagers with ADHD acquire useful coping mechanisms, problem-solving skills, and the fortitude to persevere in the face of obstacles. They develop the ability to function in an environment that does not always meet their demands, and this resiliency can be useful in many facets of life.

6. *High Energy Level*: Although having too much energy might be difficult to control, it can also lead to high levels of productivity and zeal. Teenagers with ADHD may be very active, participating in sports, physical activities, or other activities requiring a lot of energy and endurance. Their energy may be directed into activities that are consistent with their passions and interests.

7. <u>*Effective Multitasking and Quick Thinking:*</u> ADHD often helps people multitask well and think quickly. Teenagers with ADHD can multitask, change directions quickly, and adjust to changing circumstances. Fast-paced surroundings and circumstances that call for adaptability may benefit from this mental agility and multitasking.

8. <u>*Empathy and Sensitivity*</u>: Teenagers with ADHD often have an enhanced capacity for empathy and sensitivity. They often exhibit compassion and empathy by being sensitive to the needs and feelings of others. The development of helpful and welcoming social environments may be facilitated by this emotional intelligence.

9. <u>*Entrepreneurial Spirit*</u>: Teenagers with ADHD often exhibit creative, unconventional thinking, and energy, which might support an entrepreneurial attitude.

They could naturally be drawn to taking chances, seizing fresh possibilities, and choosing unorthodox routes to success.

Teenagers with ADHD may develop a good self-image, gain resilience, and make the most of their special talents by embracing and fostering their potential and skills. Recognizing their talents and offering help based on their requirements may enable them to achieve academic, artistic, and social success. Teenagers with ADHD may significantly contribute to society and enjoy successful, satisfying lives with the correct support and chances.

CHAPTER 2: NAVIGATING THE ADOLESCENT BRAIN

Developmental Changes and ADHD

Neurodevelopmental disorder Attention Deficit Hyperactivity Disorder (ADHD) affects people of all ages, including kids and teenagers. For those who have ADHD, the interplay between the disorder and the developmental changes that take place during these formative years may have a big influence. For effective support and therapies, it is essential to understand how these developmental changes and ADHD interact. Let's look at several major areas where developmental changes might affect how ADHD manifests and is treated in kids and teenagers:

1. *Executive Functioning*: During infancy and adolescence, there is tremendous growth in executive functions, which include abilities like organization, planning, and impulse control. But those who have ADHD often have delays or deficiencies in these areas. During these developmental phases, the problems brought on by ADHD, such as issues with attention, organization, and self-regulation, might be more noticeable. Children and adolescents with ADHD may progressively improve these abilities with the use of tailored therapies and education on the developmental delay in executive functioning.

2. *Academic expectations*: As kids go from elementary to middle to high school, the expectations for their academic performance considerably rise. They must handle several topics, challenging tasks, and lengthy projects.

For those who have ADHD, these difficulties may be more problematic since they may have trouble staying organized, managing their time, and maintaining attention. The effect of ADIID on academic performance may be lessened by recognizing the higher academic demands and offering assistance, such as study skills instruction, organizational methods, and accommodations.

3. *Social Interactions*: During childhood and adolescence, social growth is essential. As kids become older, they learn to be more self-reliant, make friends, and negotiate complicated social dynamics. However, those with ADHD could have particular difficulties here. Due to their difficulties with impulse control, mood regulation, and social skills, children and adolescents with ADHD may find it difficult to establish and sustain lasting relationships.

Healthy social development may be facilitated by recognizing the social difficulties that come with ADHD and by offering social skill training and assistance.

4. *Peer contacts*: During adolescence, peer contacts become more important. Due to their impulsive conduct, lack of impulse control, and problems reading social signs, adolescents with ADHD may have extra difficulties in peer interactions. These elements may play a role in social rejection, loneliness, and poor self-esteem. Positive social development may be supported by recognizing how ADHD affects peer relationships and by creating inclusive settings that encourage understanding, empathy, and acceptance.

5. *Emotional management*: During childhood and adolescence, emotional management is a crucial component of growth.

However, those who have ADHD often struggle to successfully manage their emotions. They could have difficulty controlling their responses, impulsive conduct, and strong emotional reactions. Emotional management may become more difficult throughout adolescence due to hormonal and neurological changes. Adolescents with ADHD may handle these changes more successfully if their emotional needs are acknowledged, and they are given support, coping mechanisms, and access to therapy, and their emotional needs are acknowledged.

6. _Independence and Responsibility_: The adolescent years are characterized by a rise in independence and accountability. Due to issues with organization, time management, and executive functioning, adolescents with ADHD may have extra problems while assuming these duties.

Teenagers with ADHD may progressively improve these abilities by understanding how ADHD affects independence and responsibility and by offering direction, structure, and support.

To best meet the unique requirements of children and adolescents, therapies and support must take into account the relationship between ADHD and developmental changes. Understanding the difficulties brought on by ADHD during these formative years enables focused therapies that may enhance functioning overall, social development, emotional well-being, and academic performance. Individuals with ADHD may negotiate developmental changes more skillfully and realize their full potential by giving the appropriate support, direction, and accommodations.

Executive Functioning and Impulsivity

A group of cognitive processes known as executive functioning are in charge of regulating, controlling, and managing our thoughts, activities, and behaviors. These processes are essential for carrying out everyday activities including organizing, planning, solving problems, making decisions, and self-control. However, people with ADHD often have deficits in executive functioning, which may show up as issues with organization, concentration, and impulse control. Particularly, impulsivity is a typical trait linked to ADHD and may have a big influence on how someone functions and lives their everyday life. Let's investigate the connection between impulsivity and executive performance in the setting of ADHD:

1. *Attention and Impulsivity*: Executive functioning depends heavily on attention, and people with ADHD often have trouble maintaining it. On the other hand, impulsivity entails doing an action without giving it much thought or taking the results into account. Impulsivity may show up in people with ADHD as a struggle to control improper reactions or behaviors. They could speak hurriedly, interrupt others, or make snap judgments. Due to their difficulty controlling their attention, people with ADHD are more likely to act on impulses without thinking through the implications or considering other options. This leads to impulsive actions.

2. *Impulsivity and Self-Control:* Self-control is yet another essential component of executive function. It requires the capacity to control one's emotions, withstand temptations, and postpone fulfillment.

Impulsive actions are often a result of self-control issues in ADHD sufferers. They could struggle to manage emotional outbursts, wait their time, or refuse quick rewards. The difficulties with self-control and impulsivity may have an impact on a person's ability to succeed academically, engage with others, and operate as a whole.

3. _Planning and Organization_: Planning and organization problems, in particular, may affect executive functioning and lead to impulsive actions. It is difficult to build organized plans, divide work into manageable segments, and establish priorities when there are problems in these areas. As a result, people with ADHD may have trouble making impulsive decisions because they tend to act on their immediate wishes or possibilities without fully weighing all of their options or contemplating the long-term effects.

4. _reaction Inhibition_: The capacity to suppress or inhibit an instinctive or prepotent reaction. It is essential for reining in impulsive conduct. People with ADHD often struggle with reaction inhibition, which leads to impulsive behavior. They could struggle to think things through before acting, to control impulsive speech or conduct, or to contemplate the possible effects of their actions.

5. _Time Management_: Planning, prioritizing, and effectively finishing activities all depend on effective time management, which is directly related to executive functioning. People with ADHD often suffer from time management skills, finding it challenging to accurately predict and allot time. This may encourage impulsive behaviors like procrastinating, rushing through work, or disregarding the amount of time needed to do tasks.

ADHD Treatment: Addressing Impulsivity and Improving Executive Functioning

Implementing interventions to address these issues in people with ADHD requires an understanding of the connection between executive functioning impairments and impulsivity. The following strategies might be useful:

1. _Behavioral therapies_: Impulsivity and executive functioning issues in ADHD patients may be addressed with behavioral therapies. These interventions might include the use of regular routines, the division of work into smaller, more manageable phases, the use of visual aids and reminders, and the communication of precise expectations and guidelines. Promoting self-control and minimizing impulsive behaviors may also be accomplished with the use of reward systems and constructive criticism.

2. <u>*Cognitive-Behavioral Therapy (CBT):*</u> CBT may help with impulsive issues and can enhance executive functioning abilities. CBT procedures work to improve problem-solving and decision-making abilities by raising awareness of impulsive thoughts and actions, creating strategies for impulse control, challenging automatic responses, and more. Through CBT, people with ADHD may discover their impulsive tendencies and gain coping skills to control them.

3. <u>*Medication*</u>: In certain circumstances, a doctor may recommend medication to assist control the symptoms of ADHD, such as impulsivity and issues with executive functioning. The executive functioning of the brain may be enhanced by stimulant drugs like methylphenidate or amphetamines. Impulsivity and executive functioning issues may also be treated with non-stimulant drugs like atomoxetine.

4. _Skill-Building therapies_: People with ADHD may enhance their executive functioning skills with targeted skill-building therapies. These treatments could include teaching time management skills, self-monitoring tactics, planning and organizing approaches, and problem-solving abilities. Individuals with ADHD may better control impulsive behaviors and enhance overall functioning by developing their executive functioning abilities.

5. _Environmental Modifications_: Making changes to the environment may help people with ADHD better control their impulsive and executive functioning difficulties. This may include arranging and structuring the physical environment, reducing outside distractions, establishing reliable routines, and using visual signals and reminders.

Environmental changes may enhance executive functioning generally, assist people with ADHD maintain attention, and lessen impulsive behavior.

6. *Supportive Networks*: People with ADHD need to create a network of loved ones, friends, instructors, and medical experts. The support network may provide direction, understanding, and encouragement by being aware of the difficulties brought on by impulsivity and executive functioning. This network may assist people with ADHD in creating solutions, reinforcing good behaviors, and providing a secure setting for talking about and managing issues connected to impulsivity.

People with ADHD may enhance their social relationships, academic achievement, and general quality of life by treating impulsivity and improving executive functioning abilities.

To successfully manage impulsivity and promote executive functioning in people with ADHD, it is crucial to adopt a comprehensive strategy that combines behavioral interventions, therapy, medication (when appropriate), skill-building interventions, environmental modifications, and a supportive network.

Managing emotions and exercising self-control

Self-control and emotional regulation are crucial abilities that allow people to successfully regulate their emotions, urges, and actions. They are crucial to relationships, decision-making, and general well-being, among other facets of existence. Emotional regulation and self-control, however, may be extremely difficult for many people, including those with ADHD or other neurodevelopmental problems.

Techniques for Improving Emotional Control and Self-Regulation

1. *Increasing Emotional Awareness*: Emotional control success begins with increased emotional awareness. People who are encouraged to name and classify their emotions are better able to discern emotional triggers and states. This may be accomplished by participating in mindfulness exercises, writing, or having candid conversations about feelings. Emotional awareness may be supported by developing emotional language and educating people about the bodily experiences connected to various emotions.

2. *Putting Coping Strategies into Practice*: Giving people coping skills may help them better control their emotions and behaviors. Deep breathing techniques, gradual muscular relaxation, exercise, mindfulness activities, and meditation are a few examples of these methods.

Promoting the use of constructive self-talk and reshaping unfavorable beliefs may both aid in the development of emotional control and self-control.

3. *Establishing a Supportive Environment*: Promoting emotional regulation requires the creation of a supportive environment that recognizes and validates feelings. Creating a secure environment where people may express their emotions without fear of retaliation or condemnation encourages healthy emotional expression and growth. Being around others who are in supportive relationships, such as family, friends, or therapists, may provide direction and encouragement for learning how to regulate one's emotions.

4. *Developing Problem-Solving Skills*: Problem-solving abilities are essential for controlling difficult circumstances and emotions.

It is possible to improve someone's ability to regulate themselves by teaching them how to recognize difficulties, come up with potential solutions, weigh the pros and cons, and make well-informed judgments. Encouragement of a methodical and logical approach to problem-solving aids people in thinking through the consequences of impulsive acts and aids them in making more deliberate decisions.

5. *Engaging in Self-Reflection and Mindfulness Practices:* Mindfulness techniques foster present-moment awareness, non-judgment, and acceptance of emotions. People may learn to manage their emotions and gain self-discipline by practicing mindfulness techniques like body scans and guided meditation. People may monitor their emotional states, assess their self-control efforts, and establish objectives for growth via self-reflection activities like journaling or routine self-assessment.

6. _Seeking Professional Support_: In certain circumstances, receiving professional assistance, such as therapy or counseling, may help enhance one's capacity for self-discipline and emotional control.

Therapists may provide direction, impart specialized techniques, and assist people in overcoming emotional difficulties. Both dialectical behavior therapy (DBT) and cognitive-behavioral therapy (CBT) place a strong emphasis on teaching clients how to manage their emotions. It takes time, effort, and encouragement to improve emotional control and self-control. People may improve their ability to control their emotions, make wise choices, and foster healthier relationships by putting these skills development tactics into practice.

Individuals may be empowered to handle life's problems with resiliency and success by being made aware of how important emotional regulation and self-control are, as well as by being given the appropriate resources and support.

PART II: BUILDING A SUPPORTIVE FOUNDATION

CHAPTER 3: FOSTERING OPEN COMMUNICATION

Creating a Safe and Trusting Environment

People can only flourish, develop, and feel confident in their interactions and relationships in a safe and trustworthy atmosphere. Establishing an atmosphere that values safety and trust, whether at home, in learning environments, or the community, supports emotional health, wholesome relationships, and general development. Let's examine the significance of cultivating a secure and dependable atmosphere and methods for doing so:

1. *Psychological Safety*: A psychologically safe atmosphere is one in which people may express their views, ideas, and feelings without worrying about criticism or retaliation. It enables risk-taking flexibility, open communication, and teamwork. People are more willing to express their opinions, participate in thoughtful debates, and give back to the community or organization when they feel psychologically secure.

2. *Emotional Support*: Establishing a secure and dependable environment requires the provision of emotional support. This entails paying attention to what people are saying, demonstrating empathy and understanding, and validating their feelings. An environment of trust and acceptance is fostered through promoting free communication and giving people the chance to express their emotions.

3. _Respect and Non-Judgement_: Respect and non-judgment are essential for creating a secure and dependable atmosphere. It entails accepting variety, appreciating unique qualities, and encouraging inclusion. Individuals are more willing to participate, contribute, and establish genuine relationships with others when they feel valued and accepted for who they are.

4. _Effective and Clear Communication_: A foundational element of a secure and reliable environment is effective and clear communication. It entails speaking truthfully and freely about ideas and expectations, engaging in active listening, and fostering open communication. It's easier to establish a feeling of stability and predictability when there are defined rules, limits, and expectations.

5.   *Promoting Collaboration and Cooperation*: Collaboration and cooperation provide a community or group members with a feeling of oneness and belonging. A secure atmosphere where people feel valued and supported is created by fostering cooperation, shared decision-making, and appreciation for all viewpoints. People gain confidence in their community and peers by encouraging a feeling of shared accountability and objectives.

6. *Setting Clear Boundaries and Safety Measures*: Boundaries and safety measures must be set in place for one's physical and mental well-being. This might include establishing standards for acceptable conduct, enforcing rules against harassment and bullying, and putting safety procedures into place. In order to maintain a safe and trustworthy atmosphere, it is important to prioritize each person's bodily and emotional safety.

7. <u>*Reliability and Consistency*</u>: Reliability and consistency in actions and reactions help to foster a feeling of security and confidence. Trust is built within a community through consistently preserving beliefs, keeping promises, and being dependable in assisting others. People feel safer and more at ease participating in the environment when they can count on others to be reliable and consistent.

8. <u>*Creating Relationships and ties*</u>: Fostering relationships and ties throughout the community helps people feel secure and trusted. People create supportive connections more easily when chances for social engagement, team-building exercises, and a feeling of belonging are provided. These relationships provide a network of support that promotes emotional stability and a feeling of security.

It takes constant work and care to maintain a secure and trustworthy environment. It entails encouraging cooperation, respectful dialogue, emotional support, and open communication. Individuals' needs and well-being may be prioritized in order to create a secure and trustworthy atmosphere that fosters personal development, wholesome relationships, and a sense of community for everyone involved.

Active Listening with Empathy

Empathy and active listening are crucial traits that promote clear communication, mutual understanding, and deep relationships between people. These abilities are very helpful in forging lasting bonds, settling disputes, and fostering a positive atmosphere. Let's examine the significance of active listening and empathy as well as methods for developing these abilities:

1. _Active Listening_: Active listening goes beyond just hearing words and is a focused, purposeful style of listening. It is listening intently to the speaker, observing verbal and nonverbal signs, and making an effort to comprehend what they are trying to say. Focus, endurance, and an open mind are necessary for active listening. People may show respect, validate other people's experiences, and promote good communication by actively listening to them.

- Active listening techniques: - Give the speaker your undivided attention by blocking out all other noise.

- Keep eye contact: Show that you are paying attention and that you are present.

- Refrain from interjecting: Give the speaker a chance to finish their point without being interrupted.

- Consider what has been said: To guarantee comprehension, summarize or paraphrase the speaker's message.

- Request clarification: For a better grasp of the speaker's viewpoint, ask for clarification.

- Demonstrate nonverbal clues Your involvement may be shown by nodding, grinning, and making supportive motions.

- Exercise patience by giving the other person a chance to finish their thought before answering.

2. *Empathy*: The capacity to comprehend and relate to the emotions, ideas, and experiences of another is known as empathy. It entails placing oneself in another person's position, reserving judgment, and demonstrating compassion. Empathy enables people to relate to one another emotionally, validate the feelings of others, and provide a sense of support and understanding.

- Practice perspective-taking by attempting to comprehend the issue from the viewpoint of the other person as one of the strategies for developing empathy.

- Listen without passing judgment: Establish a secure environment where people may express themselves without worrying about being judged.

- Appreciate feelings: Even if you don't have the same viewpoint as them, acknowledge and respect other people's feelings.

- Exhibit sincere interest: Show genuine interest in and a desire to comprehend the experiences of the other person.

- Exercise your active imagination by putting yourself in comparable circumstances to better understand how others feel.

- Exercise empathy through conversation: Develop empathy in a variety of situations, including those involving friends, family, coworkers, and strangers.

- Offer assistance: By providing support, consolation, or encouragement to people in need, you may demonstrate empathy.

Benefits of Empathy and Active Listening

1. _Improved Communication_: By promoting comprehension, clarity, and trust, active listening and empathy enhance communication. People are more willing to express themselves honestly and freely when they feel heard and understood.

2. _Conflict Resolution_: Effective conflict resolution requires active listening and empathy. People may establish common ground, explore alternatives, and create mutually beneficial outcomes by listening intently and empathizing with one another's viewpoints.

3. _Deeper ties and Stronger partnerships_: Empathy and active listening foster deeper ties and stronger partnerships. People are more likely to feel trusted, respected, and emotionally connected when they feel heard, validated, and understood.

4. _Emotional Support_: Empathy and active listening help people feel supported emotionally. In trying circumstances, people may provide solace, validation, and confidence by sincerely listening and empathizing with them.

5. _Personal Growth_: Active listening and empathy-building techniques help people grow personally by broadening their horizons, fostering patience and understanding, and improving emotional intelligence.

Individuals may develop meaningful relationships, enhance communication, and create a supportive and empathic atmosphere by engaging in active listening and empathy. These abilities not only help people in their interpersonal relationships but also promote peaceful interactions in the workplace, in educational settings, and communities at large.

Encouraging Honest Dialogue

Effective communication, the development of trust, and the promotion of interpersonal understanding all depend on honest conversation. It encourages honest and open discussion of issues, worries, and viewpoints, resulting in beneficial connections and positive results. It's critical to foster open communication in a variety of situations, including interpersonal relationships, businesses, educational institutions, and community activities. Let's examine the significance of open communication and methods for encouraging it:

1. *Appreciating Diverse Perspectives*: Promoting open discussion requires appreciating and respecting other viewpoints. It provides a comfortable environment for people to express themselves freely when it is acknowledged that everyone contributes their own

experiences and ideas to the discourse. Stressing the value of other points of view helps in removing obstacles and fosters a workplace that is more inclusive and collaborative.

2. _Active Listening_: Promoting open communication requires active listening. It is giving the speaker your complete attention, listening carefully to what they have to say, and expressing a sincere desire to comprehend their viewpoint. People who actively listen to others demonstrate respect, affirm their experiences, and provide the groundwork for frank and open dialogue.

3. _Suspending Judgment_: It's important to suspend judgment and enter talks with an open mind to promote open communication. When people feel evaluated or ridiculed, they can be reluctant to express their opinions openly.

It is possible to freely express ideas, encourage others to speak out and foster an environment of openness and trust by creating a nonjudgmental atmosphere.

4. _Establishing Psychological Safety_: Establishing psychological safety is essential for promoting open communication. It entails creating a setting where people feel free to voice their ideas, worries, and even divergent beliefs without fear of repercussions. Individuals might feel more comfortable being open and vulnerable in conversation by developing trust and ensuring secrecy.

5. _Giving Constructive Feedback_: Honest communication requires constructive criticism. It entails providing criticism courteously and helpfully, emphasizing the behavior or ideas rather than criticizing the person.

People are inspired to have open conversations and share knowledge when you give them criticism that is precise, practical, and geared toward progress.

6. _Promoting Curiosity and Questioning_: Promoting curiosity and questioning encourages people to engage in open discussion. As a result, interactions become deeper and more meaningful. Curiosity encourages a desire to learn about and comprehend all viewpoints. People may investigate concepts, refute presumptions, and develop deeper insights by asking questions and encouraging others to do the same.

7. _Positively Handling Conflict_: While conflict is a normal component of human relationships, how it is handled may have a big influence on how open and honest a discussion is.

Encouragement of open, courteous, and constructive conflict resolution helps avoid misconceptions and promotes the settlement of problems via direct, open conversation. During confrontations, teaching conflict resolution techniques and encouraging active listening may result in fruitful and sincere dialogues.

8. _Set an Example_: Setting an example as a leader or facilitator is essential to promoting open communication. Encourage others to do the same by practicing active listening, courteous dialogue, and openness to other points of view. People are more inclined to have honest talks when they see the value and significance of open communication.

Individuals may develop better connections, increase understanding, and come up with innovative solutions by promoting open communication.

Sincere conversation fosters a climate of mutual respect, trust, and cooperation, which has favorable effects in both personal and professional contexts. People can only fully connect, learn from one another, and strive toward their development and advancement via honest and open conversation.

CHAPTER 4: STRENGTHENING RELATIONSHIPS

Parent-Teenager Bonding

The link between parents and teenagers is special and transforming, and it is essential to adolescents' emotional growth and well-being. Teenagers need to feel loved and supported to develop, feel confident in themselves, and be happy in general. To help them deal with the difficulties and changes of adolescence, it offers a solid foundation of support and direction. Let's talk about the value of developing strong bonds between parents and teenagers and discuss methods for doing so:

1. *Honest and Open Communication*: Establishing honest and open communication is essential for forging a solid link between parents and teenagers. Teenagers may share their ideas, worries, and emotions safely when discourse, active listening, and nonjudgmental talks are encouraged. Parents' relationships with their teenagers are strengthened when they encourage open conversation so that they may comprehend their opinions and experiences.

2. *Quality Time*: Strengthening the link between parents and teenagers may be achieved by spending quality time together. Shared interests, hobbies, and activities promote a feeling of community and provide enduring memories.

Setting aside time to connect with teens shows concern and interest in their life, whether it's via meaningful talks, playing games, cooking together, or just going for walks or playing games.

3. *Empathy and Understanding*: Establishing a solid link between parents and teenagers requires demonstrating empathy and understanding. The teenage years may be a difficult period marked by emotional ups and downs. Parents may build a relationship of trust and compassion with their children by understanding their experiences, acknowledging their feelings, and providing assistance. Teenagers are more likely to turn to their parents for advice and emotional assistance as a result of this feeling of security.

4. *Respect limits*: Respecting limits is essential to preserving a strong relationship between parents and teenagers.

Teenagers are forming their identities and desiring independence, so it's crucial to acknowledge and accept that urge. Teenagers are more likely to feel trusted and respected in a relationship if they are encouraged to voice their thoughts, make choices, and accept responsibility for their actions.

5. *Participatory Decision*: Making Teenagers might have a sense of empowerment and worth when they participate in decision-making processes. Giving kids a say in family decisions, such as making rules, organizing events, or talking about chores, fosters their feeling of ownership and deepens their relationship with their parents. Within the family dynamic, collaborative decision-making fosters a feeling of collaboration and respect for one another.

6.   _Positive   Reinforcement_: Offering encouragement and positive feedback may help build a strong link between parents and adolescent children. Teenagers' self-confidence and their bond with their parents are both boosted when their efforts, accomplishments, and progress are acknowledged. A loving and encouraging atmosphere that fosters a strong parent-teenager relationship is created by acknowledging their accomplishments and giving them words of encouragement.

7. _Emotional Support_: Because adolescence may be an emotionally turbulent period, it's important to provide emotional support to develop a solid relationship. Teenagers may negotiate problems and build resilience by having adults who are accessible to listen, provide assistance, and provide a secure environment for them to express their feelings.

Teenagers may feel understood and supported when others are empathic, validate their emotions, and provide assurance.

8. *Set a Good Example*: Parents act as role models for their children, and setting a good example is essential to forging a solid relationship between parents and teens. Teenagers have a good example to follow when adults act with respect, honesty, compassion, and efficient communication. Parents who provide an example of positive attitudes and actions for their children help them build emotional intelligence as well as their relationship.

An effective parent-teenager relationship involves work, patience, and understanding. Parents may develop an atmosphere that is loving and supportive for their adolescent children by encouraging open communication, spending quality time with them, demonstrating empathy, and respecting their limits. A strong relationship between a parent and an adolescents' general well-being and development are enhanced as they travel the thrilling and changing path of adolescence on a foundation of trust, support, and love.

Sibling Dynamics and ADHD

When one or more siblings have ADHD (Attention-Deficit/Hyperactivity Disorder), it may add another level of dynamics and difficulties to the already complicated and distinctive sibling relationships. ADHD is a neurodevelopmental condition that impairs attention, impulsivity, and hyperactivity. It may hurt the family unit, particularly sibling relationships. To provide a caring and supportive atmosphere, it's critical to comprehend how siblings connect and interact when one has ADHD. Let's examine the interactions between siblings, ADHD, and relationship-building techniques:

1. Having a basic awareness of ADHD is important for siblings to appreciate the condition and its impact. Siblings may grow in empathy, compassion, and tolerance for their ADHD sibling by learning about the disorder. Siblings may avoid misunderstandings and cultivate a more supportive attitude by realizing that ADHD is a neurological illness rather than a decision.

2. *Fostering Open Communication*: Siblings must communicate openly to comprehend one another's needs and emotions. Fostering understanding and support among siblings involves creating a secure area where they may voice their ideas, worries, and frustrations with ADHD. Such open communication might be facilitated by regular family gatherings or sibling bonding activities.

3. *Teaching Siblings About ADHD*: Teaching siblings about ADHD will help them better understand the difficulties their sibling confronts. Age-appropriate books, articles, or films regarding ADHD may provide explanations of the disease and aid siblings in understanding their sibling's experiences. This understanding may increase empathy and lessen sentiments of annoyance or anger.

4. Siblings without ADHD should get equal attention and individualized assistance, thus parents must make sure of this. All siblings must get equal attention and time, even if the sibling with ADHD may need more help and adjustments. A balanced and inclusive family atmosphere may be created by celebrating individual successes and abilities.

5.   *Promoting Collaboration and Teamwork*: Siblings may assist one another by encouraging a spirit of collaboration and teamwork. Sibling collaboration on tasks, hobbies, or projects may foster understanding and cooperation. Siblings may respect one other's abilities, work well together, and foster a feeling of camaraderie thanks to this shared experience.

6. *Handling Sibling Rivalry*: When one sibling has ADHD, managing sibling rivalry might be more difficult. Parents may be very helpful in resolving disputes and promoting justice. Rivalry may be reduced and a more harmonious sibling relationship can be fostered by setting clear expectations, creating consistent standards, and constructively resolving problems.

7. *Promoting Empathy and Support*: Fostering empathy and support among siblings is essential to creating a harmonious relationship.

Encourage siblings to help and encourage one another, especially during trying times. Simple acts of kindness, like assisting with chores or speaking encouraging words, may go a long way toward fostering supportive relationships between siblings.

8. *Sibling Bonding Activities*: Taking part in sibling bonding activities may improve the link between siblings, including those who are ADHD-affected. Games, hobbies, and family excursions are examples of activities that may foster a feeling of connection and happy memories. These activities provide siblings with the chance to interact, have fun, and establish a solid support system.

It's crucial to understand that every family and sibling relationship is different, and addressing ADHD dynamics may need different approaches. Seeking advice from mental health specialists may provide extra methods and support for handling sibling interactions.

These professionals can include therapists or support groups that specialize in ADHD. Parents may encourage healthy sibling relationships and create an atmosphere where all siblings, including those affected by ADHD, can flourish by encouraging understanding, empathy, and support.

PART III: ACADEMIC SUCCESS AND SKILL DEVELOPMENT

CHAPTER 5: MANAGING SCHOOL CHALLENGES

Collaborating with Teachers and Schools

Collaboration between parents, instructors, and schools is essential when an adolescent has ADHD (Attention-Deficit/Hyperactivity Disorder) to provide the required assistance and provide an inclusive learning environment. ADHD may affect a teen's social connections, academic performance, and general well-being. Together, parents and teachers can support adolescents with ADHD in achieving academic and emotional success. Let's look at the significance of working with teachers and schools to support teenagers with ADHD as well as successful cooperation techniques:

1. *Create open communication channels*: Effective teamwork requires regular, open communication. To provide information regarding their teen's ADHD diagnosis, strengths, problems, and any particular accommodations or solutions that have worked well, parents should first begin contact with teachers and schools. Teachers should also keep parents informed about their adolescent's development, difficulties, and any concerns via frequent communication.

2. <u>*Disseminate Useful Information*</u>: Parents should educate teachers fully about their teen's ADHD, including medical diagnoses, assessments, and Individualized Education Plans (IEPs) or 504 plans, if appropriate. By exchanging this information, instructors may better grasp the unique requirements of the adolescent and adjust their approach. Parents may also provide advice on practical tactics or modifications that have previously been successful.

3. <u>*Collaborate on customized Support Plans*</u>: Parents and educators may create a customized support plan for the ADHD adolescent by working together. This plan may include particular accommodations like preferred seating, more time for tasks or tests, the use of aids or devices, or altered assignments. The efficacy of the support plan depends on regular meetings to evaluate and modify it in light of the adolescent's development and shifting requirements.

4.   _Advocate for Services and Accommodations_: Parents may advocate for their adolescent's needs by working with educators and administrators to make sure the right services and accommodations are in place. This may include engaging actively in the development of the IEP or 504 plan, attending meetings, and providing documents. Collaborative advocacy ensures that the academic and social-emotional requirements of the adolescent are satisfied in the school setting.

5. _Share Information and Provide input_: Regular input from parents and instructors helps track the adolescent's development and modify treatments as necessary. Parents may discuss their teen's experiences at home, the effects of medicine, and any behavioral or functional changes. On student conduct in the classroom, social interactions, or academic achievement, teachers might provide feedback.

This information sharing encourages a comprehensive approach to assistance and identifies opportunities for improvement.

6. *Encourage the Development of Executive Functioning Abilities*: For adolescents with ADHD, collaborating with instructors to encourage the development of executive functioning abilities is essential. These abilities include self-control, planning, organization, and time management. Teachers may support students in putting these tactics into practice by giving clear instructions, segmenting projects into manageable pieces, using visual aids, and encouraging the use of planners or digital tools. Teenagers may better handle their obligations when executive functioning abilities are consistently reinforced at home and school.

7. *Promote Consistency and Structure*: Teenagers with ADHD benefit from consistency and structure.

Establish routines and consistency in the school setting by working with the instructors. Teenagers with ADHD may manage their time, tasks, and transitions more effectively throughout the school day with the support of consistent expectations, clear instructions, and visual timetables.

8. *Encourage a Supportive Learning Environment*: Parents and teachers should work together to create a welcoming and inclusive learning environment for adolescents with ADHD. This entails building an environment of acceptance and respect among peers, encouraging empathy and understanding among classmates, and teaching them about ADHD. Differentiated teaching methods that take into account various learning styles and provide chances for active participation may be used by teachers.

Always keep in mind that a successful partnership requires constant communication, adaptability, and a shared dedication to the academic and general well-being of the adolescent. By collaborating, parents and teenagers with ADHD may flourish in an atmosphere where instructors can help them discover their skills and realize their full academic and social potential.

Homework Strategies and Study Skills

Teenagers with ADHD (Attention-Deficit/Hyperactivity Disorder) may struggle with homework owing to their attentional, organizational, and time management issues. Teens with ADHD may manage their homework load and acquire important academic abilities, nevertheless, with the correct plans and study techniques.

The following techniques may help teens with ADHD complete their schoolwork and develop their study skills:

1. _Create a Consistent Homework Routine_: When it comes to handling homework, consistency is essential. By designating a certain time and location for homework each day, you may assist your adolescent in developing a reliable homework habit. This schedule will provide them with structure and encourage them to make it a habit to turn in their assignments on time.

2. _Break Tasks into Smaller, Manageable Stages_: For teens with ADHD, breaking school assignments into smaller, more manageable stages might help them seem less daunting. Help your adolescent build a to-do list by assisting them in defining the exact chores needed for each assignment. As they finish each stage, this strategy fosters a feeling of success, which lowers anxiety and increases productivity.

3. *Make Use of Visual Aids and Organizational Tools*: Teens with ADHD might benefit from using visual aids and organizational tools to keep focused and organized while doing their schoolwork. Encourage students to keep track of assignments, due dates, and significant deadlines by using tools like calendars, planners, or digital applications. They may assist prioritize activities and feel more in charge of their work by using visual reminders, checklists, and color-coding systems.

4. *Establish a Quiet Environment*: For teens with ADHD, minimizing distractions is essential to maintaining attention when completing schoolwork. Establish a distraction-free study space that is calm and clutter-free, with a minimum of technological gadgets and loud noises. If required, promote the use of noise-canceling headphones.

Teenagers may keep focused on the topic at hand by clearing the study area of extraneous distractions.

5. _Use Timers and Breaks_: ADHD makes it difficult to maintain focus for long periods. To assist your adolescent manage their time well, introduce the idea of timers and breaks. certain timer for a certain period of concentrated work, followed by a brief rest. The Pomodoro Technique, often known as time-tracking, may increase output while allowing for the required pauses to minimize mental tiredness.

6. _Teach Students Effective Study Techniques_: Teens with ADHD must learn how to effectively study. Help them identify the study techniques that suit their learning preferences.

Making study aids, summarizing knowledge in their own words, employing mnemonic devices, and using active reading methods like underlining or taking quick notes are some ways that might be useful.

7. _Promote Self-Advocacy_: Teach your adolescent how to express their needs to instructors so they can advocate for themselves. Encourage children to ask questions when they don't understand an assignment, to get further help if needed, and to talk about any adjustments they may need. They are better equipped for future academic and professional aspirations by developing self-advocacy skills.

8. _Offer Emotional Support and Encouragement_: For adolescents with ADHD, doing their schoolwork may be a cause of stress and frustration. Throughout the process, provide encouragement and emotional support.

Even for little chores, acknowledge their efforts and successes. Celebrate their victories and reassure them when they encounter difficulties. Your assistance may have a big influence on how motivated and persistent they are.

Because every adolescent is different, it could take some time for them to identify the study techniques and tactics that are most effective for them. It's crucial to engage your adolescent in the process and give them a say in picking the tactics that appeal to them. Teenagers with ADHD may overcome their homework issues and achieve higher academic performance by using these techniques and encouraging the development of excellent study habits.

Accommodations and Individualized Education Plans (IEPs)

Accessing the proper accommodations and support in the school context is essential for teens with ADHD (Attention-Deficit/Hyperactivity Disorder) to achieve academic performance and general well-being. Accommodations are changes or additions made to the curriculum or learning environment to help kids with ADHD engage in school activities more successfully. IEPs, or individualized education plans, are formalized plans that specify the particular assistance and adjustments an ADHD kid needs to succeed in the classroom. Let's look at the value of adjustments and IEPs for adolescents with ADHD and how they may help their academic journey:

1. *Individualized Support*: Each adolescent with ADHD has an IEP that is specifically tailored to match his or her requirements. These strategies consider the particular difficulties with organization, time management, impulse control, and focus. IEPs and modifications provide teens with the skills and methods required for academic achievement by focusing assistance on their unique needs.

2. *Equal Educational Opportunities*: With the use of IEPs and accommodations, teens with ADHD are given the same access to educational opportunities as other teenagers. By removing obstacles and giving students the necessary resources, these strategies level the playing field and encourage full participation in the learning process. Teenagers with ADHD may engage fully in class, complete homework, and show off their knowledge and abilities with the right accommodations in place.

3.   <u>*Individualized   Accommodations*</u>: Depending on the particular requirements of the adolescent, accommodations might take many different shapes. Preferential seating, extra time for examinations and assignments, pauses during work, the use of assistive technology, visual aids, or modified assignments are a few examples of accommodations for ADHD. Teenagers with ADHD may better control their symptoms, maintain their attention, and do tasks without unneeded barriers thanks to these adjustments.

4. <u>*Collaboration and Communication*</u>: The creation of accommodations and IEPs requires cooperation and constant communication between parents, teachers, and other educational professionals. To create a successful IEP, parents must work with the school personnel and speak out for their teen's needs.

To consistently apply accommodations and make the required adjustments to accommodate the adolescent's developing requirements, regular contact and feedback are essential.

5. _Support for Executive Functioning Skills_: For teens with ADHD, executive functioning abilities including planning, organization, and time management may be difficult. IEPs and accommodations often contain tactics and support that concentrate on these particular competencies. Schools may help teens acquire these important abilities and enhance their overall academic achievement by putting in place accommodations that promote executive functioning.

6. _Self-Advocacy and Self-Efficacy_: IEPs and accommodations may help teens with ADHD learn to advocate for themselves. Teenagers gain the ability to express their requirements, ask for assistance when required,

and take charge of their educational experience by actively engaging in the formulation and execution of their accommodations. Self-advocacy training encourages self-efficacy, self-confidence, and a feeling of control over one's academic path.

7. _Transition Planning_: IEPs also include the move from high school to either post-secondary education or a job. Goals, supports, and accommodations that get teens with ADHD ready for the next stage of their life may be included in the plan. The foundation for future success is laid through transition planning, which guarantees a seamless transfer and continuation of assistance beyond high school.

8. _Consistent Review and Evaluation_: IEPs and accommodations are not static records. To guarantee their efficacy, they are continuously examined and assessed.

To evaluate progress, pinpoint areas for development, and make necessary modifications to the accommodations and supports, parents, teachers, and other professionals engaged in the adolescent's education work together. IEPs and accommodations are effective strategies for supporting adolescents with ADHD in their academic endeavors. Accommodations and IEPs empower individuals by delivering tailored assistance, encouraging cooperation, and building self-advocacy teens to overcome obstacles, realize their academic potential and acquire the abilities required for long-term success.

CHAPTER 6: CULTIVATING EFFECTIVE STUDY HABITS

Organization and Time Management Techniques

For teens with ADHD (Attention-Deficit/Hyperactivity Disorder), planning and time management may be especially difficult. Effective study habits are crucial for academic achievement. Teenagers with ADHD may build effective study habits that optimize their productivity and academic results, nevertheless, with the correct tools and approaches. Here are some time-management and organizing tips that encourage good study habits:

1. *Keep Track of Due Dates with a Planner or Digital Calendar*: Encourage your adolescent to use a planner or digital calendar to keep track of due dates for homework, exams, and other events.

To keep on top of forthcoming chores, teach them to note crucial dates as soon as they get them and to often examine their calendar. They can visualize their workload thanks to this exercise, and they can better arrange their study time.

2. *Break Tasks into Handleable Chunks*: Teenagers with ADHD may feel overwhelmed by large tasks or projects. Teach them to divide these jobs into more manageable, smaller portions. They may avoid procrastination and experience a feeling of satisfaction as they finish each section by segmenting chores and concentrating on one step at a time.

3. *Prioritize and make a to-do list*: Assist your adolescent in ranking their chores according to the significance and due dates. Help them make a to-do list that explains the chores they must do in detail. Encourage them to prioritize tasks and give each one enough time before moving on.

The act of crossing off activities as they are finished gives people a feeling of accomplishment and spurs them on to do more.

4. _Establish Time Limits and Realistic Objectives_: Help your adolescent create time limits and realistic objectives for their study sessions. Help them identify the precise things they wish to do in a certain amount of time. Setting time restrictions for each work helps people concentrate and keeps them from spending too much time on one task at the cost of others.

5. _Establish a Distraction-Free Environment_: Effective study requires a minimal amount of interruptions. Find a place for your adolescent to study that is calm, well-lit, and free from distractions. Eliminate distractions like electronics, or promote their safe usage during scheduled breaks. Focus and concentration are easier to sustain in a supportive setting.

6. *Employ visual organizing techniques*: For adolescents with ADHD, visual organization techniques might be very beneficial. Teach children how to keep their things organized by using tools like binders or color-coded folders. Important information may be highlighted using sticky notes or visual clues. When required, visual aids make it simpler for them to find and access resources.

7. *Use the Pomodoro Technique*: This time management strategy entails working for small bursts of time while maintaining attention, followed by a break. Teach your adolescent to work for a certain amount of time—say, 25 minutes—before taking a 5-minute break. They may take a longer break after they have completed a few rounds. This method aids in sustaining focus and preventing mental tiredness.

8. *Use Study Aids and Strategies*: Work with your adolescent to determine which study aids and techniques are most effective for them. This may include strategies like active reading (highlighting, taking notes), employing mnemonics, making flashcards, or generating an original summary of the material. They may discover the best study techniques by experimenting with various strategies.

9. *Promote Self-Reflection and Evaluation*: Encourage your adolescent to make it a habit to reflect on and evaluate their academic performance. Encourage them to go back to their study sessions and note what went well and where they might have done better. They may gradually modify their study habits and methods thanks to their self-awareness.

10. *Seek Support and Guidance*: Remind your adolescent that it's OK to ask for help and direction when necessary.

Encourage them to ask their instructors, tutors, or other students for clarification or help. Stress the value of requesting assistance when confronted with problems or having trouble grasping an idea.

Remember, Since every adolescent is different, it's crucial to collaborate with them to identify the strategies that speak to them. Teenagers with ADHD may improve their learning experience, their academic achievement, and their ability to create successful study habits by putting these time management and organizing strategies into practice. These abilities will help them succeed in the future.

Enhancing Focus and Attention

Teenagers with ADHD (Attention-Deficit/Hyperactivity Disorder) may find it difficult to establish and maintain focus and attention, which are crucial cognitive abilities for scholastic performance and general productivity. Teenagers with ADHD may, however, benefit from a variety of tactics and approaches that can improve their concentration and attention. Here are a few strategies that work well to encourage concentration and focus:

1. *Reduce Distractions*: Establish a distraction-free workplace. Encourage your adolescent to study in a space that is peaceful, uncluttered, and devoid of interruptions, noise, and visual distractions. This may include switching off electronic devices or using programs that restrict access to websites or apps that are distracting during study periods.

2. *Make Use of Visual Cues*: Visual cues are potent tools for improving concentration and attention. Encourage your adolescent to highlight significant information using highlighters, sticky notes, or other visual

clues. Visual cues may help concentrate attention and enhance memory.

3. _Break activities Down Into Manageable Pieces_: Teens with ADHD may find it challenging to stay focused on large or complicated activities. Teach them to divide chores into more manageable, smaller bits. They can retain greater attention by concentrating on one step at a time and feel more accomplished as they finish each part.

4. _Set Realistic Goals and Time Limits_: Work with your adolescent to establish time limits for projects and realistic goals for study sessions. Organizing study time into concentrated chunks and allowing time for breaks helps improve concentration and reduce mental tiredness. Encourage them to follow their planned study schedule as closely as they can.

5. *Use timers or the Pomodoro Technique*: Timers may be effective time management and concentration aids. The Pomodoro Technique calls for concentrated work sessions of around 25 minutes, followed by quick breaks. Encourage your kid to set a timer, concentrate completely on their academic work until the alarm sounds, and then take a little break to refuel before continuing.

6. *Offer organized Study Plans*: Assist your adolescent in developing organized study schedules that include the objectives and activities for each study session. Organizing study time into distinct themes or topics aids concentration and attention by providing a clear road map. The structure may help you feel organized and have a plan, which helps clear your mind and improve your attention.

7. <u>*Use Multisensory Approaches*</u>: Using many senses at once will help you concentrate and pay attention. Encourage your adolescent to learn in a multimodal way by reading aloud, utilizing tactile materials, or making mind maps or visual diagrams. Their attention and recall are improved when additional senses are used throughout the learning process.

8. <u>*Include Regular Physical Activity*</u>: Research has shown that exercise helps people with ADHD improve their concentration and attention. Encourage your adolescent to include scheduled breaks for movement or exercise in their study schedule. Stretching or taking a little stroll may also help them refocus their attention and re energize their minds.

9. <u>*Practice mindfulness or meditation*</u>: Mindfulness and meditation approaches may assist teens with ADHD in improving attention, focusing more clearly,

and developing a stronger sense of self-awareness. Encourage your adolescent to engage in mindfulness practices before or during study sessions, such as deep breathing or guided meditation. These techniques may aid in mind-calming and attentional control improvement.

10. *pauses and prizes*: To keep people motivated and paying attention, provide regular pauses and prizes. Encourage your adolescent to take brief rests after finishing an activity or reaching a goal. These pauses may provide you with a mental respite and act as a motivator to keep focused and on task.

It's crucial to keep in mind that it takes time and repetition to build concentration and attention abilities. Be kind and encouraging while also recognizing your adolescent's accomplishments along the process.

You may improve their capacity to do this by putting these methods and tactics into practice, concentration, maintaining interest and achieving academic success.

Test Preparation and Exam Strategies

For kids to achieve their best academically, effective test preparation and exam methods are crucial. Implementing focused tactics may greatly improve exam performance for teens with ADHD (Attention-Deficit/Hyperactivity Disorder), who may struggle with organization, attention, and impulsivity. Here are some helpful test-taking and exam-preparation tips for assisting adolescents with ADHD:

1. Create a study timetable with your adolescent, allotting a certain amount of time for each subject or topic. It may be less stressful and minimize last-minute cramming by segmenting study time into

smaller parts. Make sure the plan is practical and permits frequent pauses to retain concentration and avoid mental tiredness.

2. *Review and Arrange Materials*: Help your adolescent to go through and arrange their study materials. Encourage them to take brief notes, underline important facts, and utilize visual aids like charts and diagrams. Exams can be more easily understood and knowledge can be more easily retrieved when the materials are organized.

3. *Engage in Active Learning*: Encourage your adolescent to use active learning strategies. This might be writing an informational summary in their own words, instructing others on a topic, or making flashcards for self-testing. Active learning encourages greater comprehension, memory retention, and material recall during tests.

4. <u>*Make Use of Memory Techniques*</u>: Encourage your adolescent to learn memory strategies that will help with test preparation. Acronyms and visual images are two examples of mnemonic techniques that may help people recall difficult material. To improve their ability to remember new information, encourage them to connect it to prior knowledge.

5. <u>*Take practice exams*</u>: Practice exams assist youngsters become used to the style and kinds of questions they can face by simulating the exam environment. Encourage your adolescent to look for practice exams, whether they are offered by instructors or are accessible online, and set aside time to complete them. Reviewing the findings might reveal areas that need further research.

6. <u>*Develop Effective Test-Taking Techniques:*</u> Teach your adolescent efficient test-taking techniques.

Before beginning the test, remind them to carefully read and comprehend the instructions. Remind them to prioritize simpler questions first to develop confidence and momentum, and to allow time depending on the importance of each question.

7. _Control Test Anxiety_: Performance might suffer from test anxiety. Encourage your adolescent to do deep breathing exercises or visualization methods to help them cope with test anxiety. Encourage them to speak to themselves positively and to be confident in their talents and preparation efforts.

8. _Exam Time Management_: Exam time management is essential. Give your child the advice to rapidly skim the whole test to determine the difficulty level and allot time appropriately. Remind them to take it slow and avoid wasting too much time on difficult questions that can slow down their performance on the test overall.

9. *<u>Maintain Focus and Avoid Distractions</u>*: Tell your adolescent to stay focused throughout tests. Remind them to thoroughly read the questions and highlight or underline essential terms. Avoid rushing or making snap decisions while picking replies. Encourage them to adopt tactics like hiding answer options to curb impulsive behavior.

10. *<u>Review and Double-Check</u>*: Make sure students understand how important it is to go over their answers and double-check their work before turning in a test. Encourage your adolescent to use the remaining time to check their answers to make sure they are accurate and comprehensive. Remind them to double-check any missed or incorrect questions.

11. *If necessary, seek accommodations*: Make sure the proper accommodations are in place for tests if your adolescent has an Individualized Education Plan (IEP) or 504 Plan. This can include more time, a place free from distractions, or accessibility to assistive technology. Work together with the faculty and administration to make sure the accommodations are applied correctly.

Keep in mind that every adolescent is different, therefore it's crucial to identify the techniques that suit them the most. Encourage your kid to try out these techniques, customize them to fit their requirements, and assess their efficacy. Teenagers with ADHD may approach examinations with confidence, maximize their performance, and succeed academically by establishing effective test preparation and testing techniques.

PART IV: NURTURING EMOTIONAL WELL-BEING

CHAPTER 7: BUILDING SELF-ESTEEM AND RESILIENCE

Celebrating Strengths and Accomplishments

To best help teens with ADHD (Attention-Deficit/Hyperactivity Disorder), it's critical to not only address issues but also acknowledge and celebrate their successes. Teenagers with ADHD may develop resilience, self-confidence, and a good self-image by providing for their emotional needs and celebrating their accomplishments. Here are some methods to acknowledge individuals' abilities and successes while promoting their mental health:

1. _Recognize and Celebrate Strengths_: Take the time to recognize and celebrate your adolescent's strengths. Unique abilities like inventiveness, tenacity, or the capacity to think beyond the box may be brought about by ADHD. Remind your adolescent of their innate talents and the advantages they offer to various settings by emphasizing these attributes.

2. _Honor Successes_: Whenever your adolescent fulfills a goal or anything noteworthy, honor it! Recognize their efforts and show delight in their successes, whether it's a high grade, finishing a project, or attaining a personal milestone. Verbal praise, modest prizes, or even organizing a special activity to mark their accomplishments may all be included in celebrations.

3. _Promote Self-Reflection_: Aid your adolescent in making self-reflection a habit.

Encourage them to periodically evaluate their development, progress, and accomplishments on a personal level. Ask open-ended questions to get them to think about their accomplishments, their areas of improvement, and their qualities. Their self-esteem and self-awareness are enhanced by this process.

4. _Offer Emotional Support_: Adolescence may be emotionally difficult, and ADHD can make things much more difficult. By attentively hearing their worries, validating their experiences, and creating a secure environment for them to express their emotions, you may provide your adolescent with emotional support. Inform them that you are available to help them through both their successes and challenges.

5. _Promote a Growth Mindset_: Stress to your adolescent the importance of developing skills via hard work and persistence.

Help them realize that failures are a normal part of learning and that errors may be excellent teaching tools. You may encourage resilience and the conviction that one can overcome obstacles by encouraging a growth mindset.

6. _Create Opportunities for Success_: Give your adolescent the chance to succeed. Set attainable objectives that are consistent with their skills and interests. Tasks should be broken down into manageable chunks, with assistance provided as required. They develop self-assurance and a good self-perception as a result of their successes, which might inspire them to take on new tasks.

7. _Promote Peer Support:_ Encourage your adolescent to interact with peers who may provide understanding and support. Taking part in mentoring or peer support programs may provide participants with a feeling of community and the chance to connect with

others going through similar struggles. Making good social relationships may improve their mental health and provide them with a network of support outside of the family.

8. _Teach Stress Management Skills_: Assist your adolescent in learning stress management skills to deal with difficult circumstances. Teach them methods like deep breathing exercises, mindfulness, exercise, or participating in their favorite pastimes. These methods may support their emotional control, stress reduction, and well-being maintenance.

9. _Promote Healthy Lifestyle Habits_: Maintaining a healthy lifestyle helps improve emotional well-being. Encourage your adolescent to place a high priority on regular exercise, a good diet, enough sleep, and effective coping skills.

Adopting healthy practices may enhance mood and resilience since physical and emotional well-being are strongly related.

10. _Seek Professional Support_: If your adolescent is having emotional difficulties, you may want to consider receiving professional assistance. A therapist or counselor with expertise dealing with ADHD-affected teens may provide direction, coping mechanisms, and a secure environment for them to express their feelings. Their mental health may be nurtured with the help of professional assistance.

Keep in mind that fostering each adolescent's requirements may differ, and emotional well-being is a lifelong process. Celebrating their successes and encouraging emotional well-being provide the groundwork for their general growth and assist them in overcoming any difficulties brought on by their ADHD.

You can enable your adolescent to flourish and realize their greatest potential by consistently offering support, inspiration, and understanding.

Overcoming Setbacks and Building Resilience

Teenagers with ADHD (Attention-Deficit/Hyperactivity Disorder) may have particular problems along the way. Obstacles and setbacks are a normal part of life. However, failures may be turned into opportunities for development and resilience if the proper approaches and perspectives are taken. The following strategies may assist teens with ADHD in overcoming obstacles and developing resilience:

1. *Encourage your adolescent to adopt a growth mindset*: A growth mindset emphasizes that skills and intellect can be improved through effort, practice, and

learning from errors. Help them realize that failures are not signs of failure, but rather a necessary part of growth. Encourage them to tackle difficulties with a positive and adaptable mentality and to see setbacks as learning opportunities.

2. _Encourage your adolescent to think back on failures and difficulties they have faced:_ Help them pinpoint the problem, what they can learn from it, and how they can go ahead with improvement. Encourage them to place more emphasis on the process than just the result, stressing the value of effort, resiliency, and taking lessons from failure.

3. _Set Realistic Expectations_: Teach your adolescent to hold oneself to reasonable standards. They must understand their abilities and limits since ADHD might present certain difficulties. As they advance, assist them in breaking objectives down into more manageable chunks.

Possessing a sense of success and avoiding emotions of overload or self-criticism are two benefits of having reasonable expectations.

4. *Promote Problem-Solving Techniques*: Encourage your adolescent to learn how to solve problems. Help them explore various alternatives, break down challenges into manageable pieces, and weigh possible outcomes. Encourage children to use their imaginations and to ask for assistance, support, or guidance when necessary. They may handle setbacks with a proactive and solution-focused perspective by improving problem-solving abilities.

5. *Teach Coping Skills*: Assist your adolescent in learning appropriate coping techniques for handling stress and difficulties. This may include methods like practicing mindfulness, journaling, deep breathing exercises, physical activity,

or participating in interests they find enjoyable. Encourage them to establish healthy coping mechanisms for stress and emotional processing to increase their resilience.

6. *Create a Supportive Environment*: Make your house a place where your adolescent feels safe talking about difficulties and asking for advice. Encourage direct dialogue, attentive listening, and empathy. Let them know that obstacles are a part of life and that you are there to help them overcome difficulties. They will be far more resilient if you continue to assist them.

7. Encourage resilience and tenacity by highlighting their significance in the face of failures. Encourage your adolescent to persevere despite setbacks or temporary failures.

Help them grow in their resolve and resilience by teaching them that obstacles are only hiccups that can be overcome with tenacity and a positive outlook.

8. *Seek Role Models and Inspiration*: Encourage your adolescent to look for people who might serve as inspirations or who have overcome obstacles to attain success. They may get drive, hope, and inspiration from this. Knowing that other people have conquered adversity and faced comparable challenges might give one confidence in their capacity to do so.

9. *Recognize and Celebrate Resilience*: Recognize and appreciate your adolescent's fortitude in the face of difficulties. Emphasize their efforts, tenacity, and the abilities they have gained to overcome obstacles. Recognize their improvement, no matter how modest, and reaffirm their self-assurance in their capacity to bounce back from difficulties in the future.

10. *Promote Support Networks*: Assist your adolescent in creating a network of peers, mentors, or support groups so that they may get in touch with others who have had comparable difficulties. Sharing knowledge, support, and encouragement with others may boost resilience and provide insightful tips for dealing with setbacks.

Keep in mind that developing resilience requires time and effort. Encourage your adolescent to see failures as chances for development and learning. With your help, advice, and resilient attitude, kids may learn the strategies they need to overcome obstacles and succeed in their journey with ADHD.

Promoting a Positive Self-Image

The general well-being and confidence of teens, especially those with ADHD (Attention-Deficit/Hyperactivity Disorder), depend on their having a good sense of themselves. Teenagers with ADHD may face particular difficulties, but with the correct encouragement and coping mechanisms, they may develop good self-concepts and appreciate their unique talents. Here are some strategies to encourage teens with ADHD to have a good self-image:

1. *Emphasize strengths*: Aid your adolescent in identifying and appreciating their advantages. People with ADHD often have distinctive traits like inventiveness, original thought, or tremendous energy. Remind them that everyone has a special set of skills and abilities and to explore and grow in these areas.

2. *Promote Self-Acceptance*: Teach your adolescent to accept themselves completely, including any obstacles brought on by their ADHD. Insist that their ADHD is just a part of who they are and does not diminish or limit them in any way.

Encourage self-compassion and educate them to treat themselves with kindness, praising their accomplishments.

3. _Offer Constructive Feedback_: Express constructive criticism that emphasizes development and progress rather than criticism. Advise on how to overcome difficulties and assist your adolescent in realizing that errors and failures are a necessary part of learning. You may encourage resilience and a development mentality in kids by phrasing feedback in a positive light.

4. _Promote Self-Advocacy_: Give your adolescent the tools to stand up for themselves and their demands. Teach kids how to express their abilities, obstacles, and any modifications they may need in a variety of contexts, including school or extracurricular activities.

They may develop self-confidence and take back control of their surroundings by speaking out for themselves.

5. *Promote a Supportive Environment*: Make your house a welcoming and understanding space where your adolescent feels free to express themselves. Promote direct dialogue, attentive listening, and empathy. Celebrate their accomplishments and give them comfort when things are difficult. Their sense of self and confidence may be substantially influenced by a supportive atmosphere.

6. *Set Realistic Expectations*: Aid your adolescent in establishing reasonable standards for themselves. ADHD may cause difficulties with planning, focusing, or time management. Encourage them to divide things into small chunks and acknowledge accomplishments as they occur.

Realistic expectations help people feel accomplished and eliminate emotions of inadequacy or self-doubt.

7. _Promote Self-Care_: Stress the value of self-care to your adolescent. Encourage them to place a higher priority on activities that enhance their emotional, mental, and physical health. This might include taking up a hobby, working out, practicing relaxation methods, spending time with close friends and family, or exploring one's creative side. Self-care helps people feel more valuable and promotes a better self-image.

8. _Encourage Your Teen to Form Positive Relationships_: Encourage your adolescent to form solid bonds with dependable classmates, mentors, or role models. Positive social relationships may increase self-worth, give one a feeling of community, and provide important support and understanding.

Encourage involvement in events or gatherings where individuals may meet people who have interests or life experiences.

9. _Pay Attention to Effort and Progress_: Instead of focusing simply on outcome-based metrics, pay attention to the effort and advancement your adolescent makes. Encourage children to make personal objectives for themselves and to acknowledge the efforts they take to achieve those goals. They get a feeling of pride and resiliency by recognizing their accomplishments and development.

10. _Encourage Self-Reflection and thankfulness_: Tell your adolescent to exercise self-reflection and thankfulness. Encourage them to consider their attributes, successes, and instances of resiliency. Encourage thankfulness by assisting them in recognizing the advantages of their life and the assistance they get.

These techniques encourage positive thinking and self-awareness.

Keep in mind that developing a healthy self-image is a journey that calls for tolerance, encouragement, and constant reinforcement. By encouraging acceptance of oneself, You may assist your adolescent with ADHD in strengthening their sense of self and embracing their special characteristics and potential by focusing on their strengths and creating a supportive atmosphere.

CHAPTER 8: MANAGING EMOTIONAL CHALLENGES

Understanding Emotional Dysregulation

Managing emotional challenges requires an understanding of emotional dysregulation.

Teenagers with ADHD (Attention-Deficit/Hyperactivity Disorder) may have trouble efficiently controlling and expressing their emotions, which is referred to as emotional dysregulation. These people could battle with emotional regulation, feel strong emotions, and have a hard time keeping their emotions under control. To assist teens in controlling their emotional difficulties, it is essential to comprehend emotional dysregulation. Consider the following important points:

1. *Recognizing Emotional Dysregulation*: Teenagers with ADHD may exhibit numerous forms of emotional dysregulation. They could suffer extreme mood fluctuations, difficulties settling down after being angry, irritation or outbreaks of wrath, or problems changing their emotional state.

Understanding that emotional dysregulation results from underlying neurological abnormalities can help you to distinguish it from willful misbehavior or rebellion.

2. *Neurological Factors*: Differences in brain function, especially regions involved in emotional control, are linked with ADHD. Teenagers with ADHD may struggle with impulse control, repressing emotional reactions, and attention management. These neurological variables may make it more difficult to control one's emotions and lead to emotional dysregulation.

3. *Effect on Daily Functioning*: A teen's daily life may be greatly affected by emotional dysregulation. Their interactions with friends, family, and classmates might be impacted, along with their academic progress and general well-being.

Uncontrolled emotional dysregulation may cause conflict, social problems, and higher levels of stress. To provide the right help, it is essential to comprehend this influence.

4. *Triggers and Weaknesses:* Understanding the causes and vulnerabilities of emotional dysregulation is crucial. Several circumstances, such as changes, criticism, or feeling overburdened, may cause strong emotional reactions. It's beneficial to recognize these triggers and collaborate with the adolescent to create management plans for them.

5. *Empathy and Validation*: Showing empathy for the youngster and affirming their feelings may have a big impact. Let them know that their feelings are legitimate and compliant in light of their difficulties. Even if you don't entirely get what they are going through, be supportive and understanding.

They feel heard, recognized, and less alone in their challenges when their feelings are validated.

6. *Teaching Emotional Regulation Skills*: Give adolescents with ADHD the skills and techniques they need to control their emotions. This might include using physical activity, writing, mindfulness techniques, deep breathing, or other avenues for emotional release. Encourage children to recognize their feelings and express them in constructive ways, such as by talking to a responsible adult or creating art.

7. *Establishing a Safe Space*: Teenagers need to feel comfortable expressing their feelings, therefore it's important to provide a safe and judgment-free atmosphere. Encourage open dialogue and attentive listening so that they may express their emotions without being afraid of being judged or criticized.

Making this environment comfortable promotes emotional transparency and allows for constructive emotional outpouring.

8. *Seeking Professional assistance*: Seeking professional assistance may be helpful if emotional dysregulation severely affects a teen's well-being or day-to-day functioning. The techniques and treatments they get may be customized to meet their unique requirements by mental health specialists with expertise in treating ADHD patients. Teenagers who get therapy may improve their coping methods, emotional control, and comprehension of their emotions.

9. *Working with Schools*: To establish a supportive atmosphere for teens with ADHD, it's crucial to work with teachers and other school personnel. Inform teachers about emotional dysregulation and how it affects students' behavior and academic performance.

Develop suitable supports, solutions, and accommodations together in the context of the educational environment.

10. *Promoting Self-Care*: Stress the significance of self-care to emotional health. Encourage teens to participate in leisure, stress-relieving, and self-care activities. This might be taking part in hobbies, spending time in nature, learning self-compassion, or doing things that make people happy and fulfilled.

Supporting teens with ADHD requires an understanding of emotional dysregulation while facing emotional problems. You may assist them in navigating their emotions and creating more effective coping strategies by acknowledging their challenges, expressing empathy and validating them, teaching them good emotional regulation techniques, and creating a supportive atmosphere.

Coping Strategies for Emotional Outbursts

Teenagers with ADHD (Attention-Deficit/Hyperactivity Disorder) may find it especially difficult to control their emotional outbursts. Extreme rage, frustration, or other strong emotions are sometimes expressed in these outbursts. Teenagers with ADHD may learn effective coping mechanisms to better control their emotions and lessen the frequency and severity of emotional outbursts. Here are some tactics to take into account:

1. Understanding Early Warning Signs Help youngsters recognize their early indicators of emotional discomfort. These symptoms might be physical (increased heart rate, tight muscles, etc.), and mental (changes in ideas or self-talk, anger, etc.). They may step in before emotions reach the point of an eruption by seeing these indications.

2. *Take a Break*: Tell teens to stop when they see their emotions becoming stronger. They may calm down and recover control of their emotions by leaving the scene or going to a quiet place. During the pause, you may find it helpful to take deep breaths, count to 10, or do a little mindfulness activity.

3. *Use techniques for self-control*: Teach adolescents self-control skills so they can regulate their emotions. They may change their emotional state and recover control over their emotions by engaging in deep breathing exercises, gradual muscular relaxation, or grounding activities (such as concentrating on the senses). Encourage them to consistently use these strategies even if they are not experiencing an emotional outburst.

4. Encourage teens to discover constructive methods to express their feelings by encouraging them to communicate their emotions.

Running, dancing, or playing an instrument are examples of physical pursuits that may be used as a way to let out emotions. Encouraging them to express their emotions by writing in a notebook or speaking with a dependable friend or family member might also be beneficial.

5. _Cognitive Restructuring_: Encourage adolescents to question and reframe unfavorable ideas that trigger emotional outbursts. Teach them to recognize and swap out unfavorable or unreasonable ideas with optimistic and reasonable ones. They may lessen emotional anguish and stop it from turning into an outburst by changing their viewpoint.

6. _Teach teens problem-solving techniques_: to deal with the underlying problems that lead to emotional outbursts. Assist them with identifying the issue, coming up with a few solutions, weighing the pros and drawbacks of each choice,

and selecting the best course of action. Future outbursts may be prevented by encouraging them to take the initiative to deal with the underlying issues.

7. _Create Support Networks_: Encourage teens to reach out to loved ones who can provide empathy and direction while they are experiencing emotional discomfort. Parents, teachers, mentors, and mental health professionals may all fall under this category. Having a support structure in place enables teens to regulate their emotions successfully and makes them feel acknowledged and valued.

8. _Develop Emotional Awareness_: By helping teens recognize and categorize their feelings, you may help them develop emotional awareness. Encourage them to recognize their feelings and consider the causes of those feelings.

They may convey their feelings more effectively and better comprehend their emotional experiences by learning a language for their emotions.

9. *Use Stress Reduction Strategies*: Stress may make emotional outbursts worse. Teach teens methods for reducing stress, such as frequent exercise, participating in hobbies, learning relaxation techniques, or locating calm-inducing activities. They may lessen the possibility of emotional outbursts by actively regulating their stress levels.

10. *Seek Professional assistance*: Seeking professional assistance may be helpful if a teen's emotional outbursts have a major negative effect on their well-being or ability to operate daily. Teenagers who struggle to adequately control their emotions might get specialized advice and treatments from mental health specialists.

Remember that everyone's coping mechanisms are unique, so it's crucial to collaborate with the adolescent to determine which ones are most effective for them. Teenagers with ADHD may learn healthy coping mechanisms and lessen the frequency and ferocity of emotional outbursts by using these techniques and offering ongoing support.

Anxiety and Depression in Teenagers with ADHD

Teenagers with ADHD (Attention-Deficit/Hyperactivity Disorder) sometimes struggle with other mental health issues, such as sadness and anxiety. Due to several reasons, including issues with executive functioning, social relationships, and academic performance, ADHD may raise the chance of having these diseases.

To provide the right assistance and intervention, it is essential to comprehend the connection between ADHD, anxiety, and depression. Here are some important things to think about:

1. _The co-occurrence of anxiety and depression_: Studies on teens have shown that depression, anxiety disorders, and ADHD co-occur often. According to estimates, 20% to 30% of people with ADHD may also have symptoms of sadness, and 30% to 40% of people with ADHD are thought to also experience symptoms of anxiety. Anxiety and sadness may be exacerbated by the problems brought on by ADHD, including impulsivity, difficulty in the classroom, and social issues.

2. Impact of Executive Functioning Issues: Teenagers with ADHD often have difficulties with executive functioning abilities, which are crucial for task management, thinking organization,

and mood regulation. Feelings of overload, worry, and a sensation of being always behind may be caused by difficulties with executive functioning. The chance of experiencing anxiety and depression may arise as a result of these difficulties.

3. _Academic and Social Stressors_: Adolescence is a time of major social and academic upheaval, which may be especially difficult for adolescents with ADHD. They could struggle to retain friendships, fit in socially, or do well academically. These pressures might exacerbate anxiety and feelings of inadequacy, which could set off depressive symptoms.

4. _Poor Self-Perception_: Due to their experiences with academic challenges, impulsivity, or social challenges, teenagers with ADHD may come to have a poor view of themselves.

They could think they are inadequate or that they are always failing, which can lead to poor self-esteem and raise the risk of depression.

5. _Effect on Daily Functioning_: Depression and anxiety may have a big effect on a teen's day-to-day functioning, including their social relationships, academic performance, and general well-being. Their motivation, focus, and capacity to participate in activities they formerly loved may all be impacted by these diseases. To provide appropriate assistance and intervention, it is crucial to recognize the effect on everyday functioning.

6. _Shared Symptoms_: Some symptoms of anxiety and sadness and ADHD are shared, which may complicate diagnosis and treatment. ADHD and these mental health issues might also include symptoms including restlessness, irritability, problems focusing, and sleep disruptions.

To identify between the diseases and create an effective treatment strategy, healthcare experts must perform a complete examination.

7. _Integrated Treatment strategy_: Teenagers with ADHD often need an integrated strategy to treat their anxiety and despair. A mix of medicine, counseling, and focused interventions may be used in this. A co-occurring anxiety or depressive disorder and ADHD symptoms may both be managed with medication. Therapy may help people control their anxiety, challenge harmful thought patterns, and create healthy coping skills. Cognitive-behavioral therapy (CBT) is one kind of treatment that can do this.

8. _Supportive atmosphere_: For teens with ADHD and co-occurring anxiety or sadness, creating a supportive atmosphere is essential. Promote direct dialogue, attentive listening, and empathy.

Give them a secure environment where they may share their feelings and have their experiences validated. Support from friends, family, and teachers may be very important to someone's overall well-being.

9. _Psychoeducation_: It's crucial to educate adolescents, their families, and teachers about the connection between ADHD, anxiety, and depression. Raising awareness of the difficulties they could be facing helps lessen stigma, improve understanding, and encourage early assistance.

10. _Promoting Healthy Coping Strategies_: Encourage healthy coping strategies for controlling the symptoms of anxiety and sadness. This may include regular exercise, participating in enjoyable hobbies, learning relaxation methods, enlisting the aid of friends and family, and creating reasonable objectives. Remind them that it is OK to ask for support and encourage them to seek professional assistance when necessary.

It's crucial to keep in mind that every adolescent has a different experience with ADHD, anxiety, and depression. Working together with educators, mental health specialists, and a support system may help give the essential assistance and intervention to assist youngsters in successfully managing these problems.

PART V: EMPOWERING INDEPENDENCE AND FUTURE SUCCESS

CHAPTER 9: TRANSITIONING TO ADULTHOOD

Developing Independence Skills

For teens, especially those with ADHD (Attention-Deficit/Hyperactivity Disorder), fostering independence is a top priority. In addition to preparing children for future success, developing independent skills also improves their sense of self-worth, self-reliance, and general well-being. The following are some methods for encouraging independence in adolescents with ADHD:

1. <u>*Self-Awareness and Self-Advocacy*</u>: Encourage teens to reflect on their strengths, struggles, and ADHD-related needs to help them become more self-aware. Teach children to speak up for themselves by expressing their needs and requesting the right help. This entails interacting with educators, expressing their choices, and contributing actively to debates regarding their upbringing and care.

2. <u>*Goal Setting and Planning*</u>: Assist youngsters in formulating both short- and long-term objectives. Larger objectives should be broken down into more manageable chunks. Teach them how to make calendars and action plans to accomplish their goals. Teenagers get a feeling of purpose and improve their organization and attention by learning to create objectives and make plans in advance.

3. _Time Management_: Independence requires effective time management. Teach teens time management techniques including making to-do lists, utilizing planners or calendars, and setting reminders. Encourage them to set priorities, set aside time for different pursuits, and divide more difficult jobs into smaller, more manageable components.

4. _Organizational Skills_: Assist teens in becoming more organized so they can keep track of their schedules, coursework, and possessions. This involves instructing them on how to create a file system, utilize folders or binders, and have a tidy workstation. Set up routines for things like handling their possessions, packing their bags, and getting ready for the following day.

5. _Problem-Solving Skills_: Aid teens in acquiring these abilities, which are necessary for conquering obstacles on their own.

Encourage them to recognize issues, come up with solutions, weigh the advantages and disadvantages of each choice, and come to wise judgments. Teenagers with strong problem-solving abilities are more resilient and capable of overcoming challenges.

6. Help teens improve their decision-making abilities by teaching them how to acquire information, analyze alternatives, take into account consequences, and make decisions that are consistent with their objectives and beliefs. Encourage them to assess the possible outcomes and take lessons from both successful and unsuccessful experiences.

7. Introduce teens to fundamental concepts in financial literacy, such as setting up a budget, saving money, and making wise financial choices. Make sure they understand the value of money, how to manage allowances or part-time income,

and the significance of creating financial goals. They can make wise selections and handle their resources properly if they acquire financial independence abilities.

8. _Life Skills_: Assist youth in learning independence-promoting practical life skills including cooking, laundry, simple housework, and personal hygiene. Providing children with these skills progressively helps them to confidently take care of themselves and their living space.

9. Support teens in developing social skills including active listening, effective communication, and dispute resolution. 9. Social Skills and Peer Relationships. Encourage them to go out and about, join groups or organizations that are relevant to their interests, and cultivate positive peer connections. Strong social abilities help people feel like they belong and are generally happy.

10. *Gradual Autonomy*: Allow teens to practice autonomy gradually. Give children the freedom to assume age-appropriate tasks and make choices within secure parameters. Gradually boosting their independence helps children become more self-assured and gets them ready for the rigors of adulthood.

Throughout this procedure, don't forget to provide direction, encouragement, and support. Honor their development and support their efforts. Each adolescent will develop independent skills gradually and at their rate. Teenagers with ADHD may acquire the abilities for future success, self-advocacy, and meaningful life through fostering independence.

CHAPTER 10: ADVOCACY AND COMMUNITY RESOURCES

Connecting with ADHD Support Groups

Joining support groups may be a very helpful way for people with ADHD (Attention-Deficit/Hyperactivity Disorder) to find understanding, direction, and encouragement. Individuals may interact with others who have similar experiences via ADHD support groups, share knowledge, and pick up coping mechanisms. Here are some major advantages of joining an ADHD support group and how to do so:

1. *Understanding and Validation*: Becoming a member of an ADHD support group may provide you with a feeling of understanding and validation. Participants may talk about their struggles, victories, and annoyances with others who have had similar experiences.

The realization that they are not alone and that many others experience the same problems as they do is a result of this validation.

2. *Peer Support and Empathy*: Support groups provide a special chance to interact with others who are facing comparable difficulties. A feeling of community is created through telling personal tales, listening to others experiences, and showing support and understanding. Participants may support one another emotionally and provide one another with helpful suggestions and coping mechanisms.

3. *Learning Possibilities*: To explore different facets of ADHD, support groups often offer educational sessions or invite guest speakers. Topics including controlling symptoms, enhancing executive function, cultivating wholesome relationships, and arguing for accommodations may be covered in these sessions.

Exchange of knowledge and learning from professionals may help people manage their ADHD more effectively.

4. *Coping Techniques and Useful Advice*: Support groups are a great place to exchange coping techniques and useful advice for handling ADHD. Members may share their own experiences, and provide advice on how to organize daily routines, time management tips, and communication skills. It might be quite beneficial to get knowledge from others who have successfully handled comparable difficulties in the past.

5. *Establishing a Support Network*: Support groups provide a chance to establish a network of people who understand the particular challenges and strengths related to ADHD. Participants can make lifelong friends, connect with mentors, and establish connections outside of group sessions.

This network offers continuing assistance and inspiration.

6. *Online Support Groups*: Online platforms provide virtual venues for people with ADHD to interact and support one another in addition to physical support groups. Online support groups provide convenience and accessibility, enabling members to communicate with one another whenever and wherever they want. These platforms may include discussion boards, chat rooms, and social media groups for ADHD support.

7. *Neighborhood Support Groups*: Look for neighborhood ADHD support groups in your neighborhood. These groups may be guided by healthcare professionals, counselors, or people with ADHD, and they can meet regularly in person or online. Local support groups provide you with the chance to engage with others in person and feel a part of your community.

8. Investigate regional, national, or worldwide organizations that are devoted to ADHD. These groups often provide resources, support groups, instructional materials, and Internet discussion forums. Examples include ADDitude magazine and CHADD (Children and Adults with Attention-Deficit/Hyperactivity Disorder), which provide access to online groups and a plethora of knowledge.

9. *Professional Advice*: For advice on reliable support groups, speak with mental health doctors or ADHD specialists. They may advise on how to locate organizations that meet certain requirements, offer suitable assistance, and maintain a secure and welcoming atmosphere.

10. *Self-Help Books and Publications*: Take a look at internet resources, self-help books, and publications that are geared toward people with ADHD.

These sites may provide insightful information, useful advice, and relatable personal stories to those in need of help. They may enhance the assistance received from support groups.

People with ADHD have the opportunity to share experiences, learn new things, and build support networks by joining ADHD support groups. Support groups provide a secure and compassionate setting where people may flourish and learn from one another, whether via physical gatherings or online networks.

Accessing Professional Services and Therapies

Accessing expert treatments and therapies is crucial for people with ADHD (Attention-Deficit/Hyperactivity Disorder) to manage symptoms, create coping mechanisms, and improve overall well-being.

These programs may provide direction, support, and customized therapies catered to the particular requirements of ADHD sufferers. Here are some essential professional services and treatments to take into account:

1. _Mental health specialists_: To diagnose and treat ADHD, specialists in mental health, such as psychiatrists, psychologists, and therapists, are essential. They can evaluate symptoms, provide treatment, and, if required, give medication. Individuals who work with mental health professionals might get specialized care plans and continuous assistance.

2. _ADHD Coaches_: Working with people with ADHD is a specialty of experts known as ADHD coaches. They provide direction, responsibility, and useful tactics for controlling symptoms and reaching individual objectives.

Executive functioning, time management, organization, and coping techniques are the main areas of attention in ADHD coaching.

3. _Cognitive-Behavioral Therapy (CBT)_: CBT is a kind of counseling that is often used to assist people with ADHD in managing their symptoms and enhancing functioning. It emphasizes recognizing and changing negative thinking patterns, creating efficient coping mechanisms, and enhancing self-control abilities. CBT may assist people with ADHD in overcoming issues with impulsivity, attention, and emotional control.

4. _Social Skills Training_: Many people with ADHD have trouble forming and maintaining connections with others. Training in social skills may help people develop their communication, perspective-taking, and social problem-solving abilities.

To improve interpersonal connections and build social competence, social skills training may be facilitated by therapists or specialized programs.

5. *Occupational Therapy (OT):* Occupational therapy may help people with ADHD perform more effectively and productively daily. The main goal of OT is to improve self-care, organization, time management, and attentional abilities. Occupational therapists collaborate with patients to create plans for controlling sensory sensitivity, enhancing motor function, and modifying settings to maximize performance.

6. *Parent Education and Training*: Parent education programs provide parents of children and teens with ADHD with information, direction, and support. These classes assist parents in understanding the particular difficulties brought on by ADHD and in learning good parenting techniques.

They provide useful methods for controlling behavior, enhancing communication, and promoting wholesome relationships.

7. *Medication Management*: For those with ADHD, medication may be an effective therapy choice. Psychiatrists or other medical experts may determine if a patient needs medicine, administer it, check on how well it works, and make any required changes. For complete ADHD care, medication management should be paired with additional therapies like counseling or coaching.

8. *Academic assistance and Accommodations*: For kids with ADHD, schools and educational institutions may provide academic assistance and adjustments. This may include more test time, preferred seating, help taking notes, or specialist training.

Working with educators and the support personnel at the school helps guarantee that people with ADHD get the assistance they need to achieve academically.

9. *Support Groups*: Joining support groups for people with ADHD may provide access to more information, new perspectives, and a feeling of community. Support groups provide a chance to interact with others going through similar circumstances, exchange stories, and pick up management techniques from one another. Support groups, whether they be online or in person, maybe a helpful addition to professional services.

10. *Vocational Services*: People with ADHD may benefit from vocational assistance with job placement, workplace adjustments, and career choices. Vocational counselors may help with career path exploration, job search skills development, and acquiring necessary accommodations at work.

Individuals might begin by speaking with their primary care physician, asking for recommendations from reliable sources, or getting in touch with neighborhood mental health groups to receive professional services and treatments. It is crucial to verify coverage and enquire about any necessary referrals or pre-authorization since insurance carriers may cover certain treatments. A procedure that is unique to each person is getting professional services and treatments. It is crucial to locate specialists in ADHD who have worked with people who have your demands in the past. With the correct assistance, people with ADHD may create useful coping mechanisms, control their symptoms, and succeed in a variety of spheres of their life.

Advocating for your Teenager's Needs

Advocating for your teen's needs when they have ADHD (Attention-Deficit/Hyperactivity Disorder) is crucial to making sure they get the help and accommodations they need to succeed. Advocacy is actively looking for and advocating tools, programs, and accommodations that will support your adolescent's academic, interpersonal, and emotional development. The following tactics will help you successfully advocate for your adolescent with ADHD:

1. *Educate Yourself*: Acquire a thorough knowledge of ADHD, its signs, and how it affects your teen's day-to-day activities. Keep up with the most recent developments in science, medicine, and educational rights. The more knowledgeable you are, the more able you will be to successfully advocate.

2. *Establish Relationships*: Create enduring connections with your adolescent's teachers, school officials, and other pertinent experts. They will be better able to grasp your teen's requirements and collaborate to create answers if they have regular contact and interaction. Keep the lines of communication open to quickly handle issues.

3. Work together with the school to develop an Individualized Education Program (IEP) or Section 504 Plan, which provides particular accommodations and support services for your adolescent. These contracts make sure that the educational requirements of your adolescent are addressed in a specific and consistent way. Encourage the use of accommodations like more test time, preferred seats, or more organizational help.

4. *Communicate Effectively*: Make sure everyone who needs to know, such as teachers, school administrators, mental health specialists, and members of the community, is aware of your adolescent's strengths, struggles, and unique needs. Give thorough details regarding their diagnosis of ADHD, pertinent medical history, and suggested treatments. Present information in a constructive, collaborative way while being aggressive and self-assured.

5. *Keep All Records*: Keep thorough notes of all interactions with your adolescent, including discussions, meetings, and significant papers. Keep a record of any correspondence—emails, letters, phone calls—you have with medical experts, educators, and other pertinent parties. These documents help demonstrate your efforts and provide background information if problems emerge.

6. Attend school meetings, such as IEP meetings, parent-teacher conferences, and school-wide planning sessions, and actively engage in them. Review pertinent papers in advance, and bring any notes or inquiries. Express your worries, provide your observations on the abilities and difficulties of your adolescent, and participate in decision-making.

7. *Be Proactive*: Foresee difficulties and deal with them before they worsen. Maintain an interest in your adolescent's academic development and maintain frequent contact with instructors to address any new issues. Actively look for tools and approaches that may help the unique requirements of your adolescent, such as tutoring or study skills courses.

8. *Promote Self-Advocacy*: Assist your adolescent in learning how to speak up for themselves and express their needs in social and academic contexts.

Teach kids about their legal rights, the best ways to express their demands, and how to get help if they need it. Encourage their self-assurance and give them the authority to take part in decision-making.

9. _Seek Outside Support_: If you have difficulties or opposition while fighting for your adolescent's needs, seek outside assistance. Consult with experts who focus on ADHD, or join parent support groups to share experiences and obtain insightful advice. These tools may provide direction and coping mechanisms for dealing with challenging circumstances.

10. _Maintain a positive attitude and be persistent:_ Advocacy may be a lengthy process, and setbacks can happen. As you speak up for your teen's needs, be upbeat, concentrated, and persistent. Celebrate little successes while being steadfast in your pursuit of your teen's best interests.

Keep in mind that successful lobbying needs endurance, tenacity, and continual dedication. You can ensure that your adolescent with ADHD has access to the services and assistance they need to realize their full potential by actively advocating for them.

concꞇusion

When your kid has ADHD, advocating for their needs is an important and continuing effort that calls for knowledge, cooperation, and perseverance. You can make sure your adolescent has the help and accommodations they need to succeed academically, socially, and emotionally by being knowledgeable about ADHD, developing strong connections with pertinent specialists, and actively participating in their school.

Successful advocacy depends on effective communication, documentation, and preventative actions. Developing your teen's self-advocacy abilities and getting outside assistance when necessary are crucial stages in enabling them to handle their difficulties and speak out for themselves. Remain optimistic, acknowledge your successes, and show resilience in the face of failure. Your advocacy work is crucial in fostering an atmosphere where your adolescent can get the services, support, and accommodations they need to succeed.

In the end, by speaking up for your teen's needs, you are promoting their self-esteem, independence, and future success in addition to assisting them in navigating their ADHD path. Your passion for standing up for your adolescent shows how much you believe in their potential and how committed you are to giving them the greatest opportunity.

Through advocacy, you may support your adolescent with ADHD in overcoming challenges, recognizing their assets, and thriving in all aspects of their life.

APPENDIX

Appendix A: Resources for ADHD Support Groups

- CHADD (Children and Adults with Attention-Deficit/Hyperactivity Disorder) - Website: www.chadd.org

- ADDitude - Website: www.additudemag.com

- National Alliance on Mental Illness (NAMI) - Website: www.nami.org

- Understood - Website: www.understood.org

- ADHD Online Support Groups - Websites and forums dedicated to ADHD support, such as Reddit's r/ADHD community (www.reddit.com/r/ADHD) or HealthBoards ADHD Forum (www.healthboards.com/boards/adhd)

Appendix B: Professional Services and Therapies

- Mental Health Professionals - Psychiatrists, psychologists, and therapists specializing in ADHD diagnosis, treatment, and therapy.

- ADHD Coaches - Professionals who provide guidance and support in managing ADHD symptoms, developing coping strategies, and achieving personal goals.

- Cognitive-Behavioral Therapy (CBT) - Therapy that focuses on modifying negative thought patterns, developing coping strategies, and improving self-regulation skills.

- Social Skills Training - Programs or therapists that help individuals with ADHD improve their communication, perspective-taking, and social problem-solving skills.

- Occupational Therapy (OT) - Therapy that assists individuals in improving daily functioning, organization, time management, and sensory and motor skills.

- Parent Training and Education - Programs that provide education, guidance, and support for parents of children and teenagers with ADHD.

- Medication Management - Consultation with psychiatrists or medical professionals to assess the need for medication and monitor its effectiveness.

- Academic Support and Accommodations - School services that provide support, accommodations, and specialized instruction to students with ADHD.

- Support Groups - In-person and online groups that offer a sense of community, support, and information sharing among individuals with ADHD.

- Vocational Services - Services that assist individuals with ADHD in exploring career options, securing job placements, and obtaining workplace accommodations.

The resources mentioned in this appendix are for informational purposes only and do not constitute an endorsement. It is important to research and evaluate each resource to determine its suitability for individual needs.